THE LAW OF ATTRACTION

A Guide on How to Apply the Law of Attraction to Your Life

Faye Froome

gain or other damages which may be caused by following the presented information in any way, shape, or form.

The following information is presented purely for informative purposes and is therefore considered universal. The information presented within is done so without a contract or any other type of assurance as to its quality or validity.

Table of Contents

Introduction

You may have heard many times before the saying "opposites attract". This could go a long way explain why some people never seem to live the life they truly desire and dream about constantly. They think every day about their dream life, and it seems wonderful. Their thoughts are always tuned into how they would like their life to change, let's face it we all do it. They envisage what their perfect reality could be like.

This goes on day after day, week after week, and year after year but nothing ever seems to change.

If this has happened to you then you may believe that opposites are drawn to each other and there is nothing you can do about it. You want "A" and all you ever realize is "B". You may work extremely hard to create the life you want to live. Sometimes you are heading in the right direction and you might even feel your life is changing, but you always seem to slide back to the same-old life you wish was at least a little bit better and you could at least see some tangible benefits but alas you don't.

This leads you entrenched into the belief that opposites are naturally going to attract to each other. After all, nobody wants to have the failure and a life going nowhere as their seemingly constant companions do they? Who would intentionally want that? So it makes perfect sense to you that whatever you wish for is never going to be a part of your reality unless somehow you win the lottery or literally strike gold but what are the odds of that happening?

Having said that though, the saying which states that opposites attract and that things will be drawn to each from other ends of the spectrum originated from the study in how to explain how electric forces interact when they are oppositely charged (Coulomb's Law, 1785).

It had nothing to do with achieving life goals, realizing dreams, and creating the perfect life you desire.

The law of attraction on the other hand says the universe will always push you towards things that have the same energy you are giving off. Like attracts like. This is the foundation of the idea that birds of a feather flock together. Things that are the same in many ways will come together.

You will have probably experienced this in one form or the other in your life already. Take your partner (if you have one) for example, you more than likely got together in the first place because you had a common attraction, either physical or intellectual.

The idea that of the law of attraction was first stated in 450 BC by Democritus (a Greek philosopher, scholar, and inventor) nearly 2,500 years ago. We will talk about its history or rather our knowledge of its existence in a later chapter, but we can mark its earliest beginnings at this point.

So ... what is it all about and can it work?

Nearly everybody's first experience of positive thoughts is always a fun thought experiment to imagine what you would do and what you would buy if you won the lottery. If you had a million dollars, where would you be right now? Maybe you would buy a beautiful home on the coast, or maybe you'd travel the world and see all the sights. Perhaps you would start your own business? Many of us have these dreams and as nice as they are, they are just that…. dreams.

So, what makes the law of attraction different?

Do you attract what you desire and deserve, or does the exact opposite happen? Can either "law" be proven or are you predisposed to a life of random acts and events? What is the history of the thought that mental focus on what you want creates the physical realization of those thoughts? What is the history behind the "likes attract" theory?

If opposites do truly attract, then why does the law of attraction say you can attract your dream life into a reality beyond your wildest dreams? If this is really the case, what steps do you have to take to start manifesting the existence you have desired for so long? Can you use this phenomenon to get fit and lose weight, become financially independent and retire early, or improve your relationships and enhance your life in other ways?

We will look at these questions in this book and try and make sense of the whole area of attracting improvements to one's life.

We dig deep into the law of attraction, something that millions of men and women say they have harnessed to finally see their dream realities appear. Let's get started by defining this life-altering characteristic of the natural world.

What Is the Law of Attraction?

The best way to define and understand anything is to listen to the people that know about the subject you are trying to get to grips with. For example, you would call an electrician when you have an electrical problem and a plumber when your water system springs a leak. They can define your problem and tell you what needs to be done to fix it or at least explain what's going on if they can't.

We are going to do the same thing here; it is probably the best place to start. There are certain people who have developed a reputation for understanding the law of attraction and how it applies to the modern world. Let's see how the law of attraction is defined by Michael J. Losier and the husband and wife team of Esther and Jerry Hicks.

Michael J. Losier

> *"You attract whatever you give your attention,*
> *energy and focus to."*

Esther and Jerry Hicks

"Like attracts like."

These law of attraction experts have all written books on the subject. Losier wrote "Law of Attraction: The Science of Attracting More of What You Want and Less of What You Don't", among other books on the subject. The Hicks team's most famous law of attraction book is "The Law of Attraction: The Basics of the Teachings of Abraham". Both are recommended as excellent sources of information on the law of attraction, authored by people who are globally respected as leaders in this field of study.

Notice how simplistic both of those definitions are.

There is not much to misunderstand here, they are just telling us how it is. By the way, natural laws are not created or invented, they just happen. They are discovered by analyzing patterns and studying large examples of data in studies completed on the subject. Losier and the Hicks did not manufacture the law of attraction, they simply discovered it at work in their lives and studied the findings.

Mr. Losier adds a little more meat on the bone to his definition by saying that you are already experiencing the law of attraction. It is always working and it's never wrong. It responds to your attention, energy, and focus, delivering the reality that is in alignment with the things you think and do.

By its very definition, you cannot become any better or worse at the law of attraction. It is simply something that is happening all the time without you even noticing, unless of course you are aware of it, which many people are not to begin with.

This can be beneficial to us. It means that once you learn proven practices to use this natural law to your advantage, you will begin realizing more of the things you want and less of the things you don't want, to paraphrase Losier.

The road to a better life through positive thoughts can be within anyone's grasp. Let us look at a simple explanation of how the law of attraction can really work.

The example that is often used at this point to describe the notion is that of giving someone a gift. When you go to give someone a gift, you will usually start by assessing what they have and what they might like. If you have a friend of humble means, who doesn't like splashing cash and who has hobbies like gardening

and reading, you will probably get them a book and some gardening gloves with a nice pattern.

Now imagine your other friend. You keep a wide range of company apparently and this person is rich. Ostentatiously so. They splash the cash all the time, they talk about their exotic holidays non-stop, they have all the latest gadgets and their home is beautiful, perfectly modern and kitted out with a ton of exciting features.

What do you buy them? They have everything. They are used to a certain standard of living. So, you probably get them theatre tickets. Or an experience day. Or a cool gadget. A beautiful watch. Providing you can afford it of course, but often you buy these gifts anyway as an attempt to please.

You get the point. The rich friend and the person who 'acts rich', gets more spent on them. They have put signals out into the universe as it were, and the universe has responded in kind. Someone who puts out humble signals and maybe does not 'act' quite so rich, ends up with a gift that is much lower in value. Which does not really make sense: surely the less rich friend would appreciate something more extravagant? Surely it would mean more to them.

This is not just about giving gifts or indeed about how you appear but just an example of how the law of attraction can work in real life.

The Birth of The Law of Attraction

As we have already stated, a law of nature has no real history. It has existed as long as the natural world has existed, such as the law of gravity. Newton was the first to define and quantify the law of gravity, but it was at work in the world long before he noticed it.

What we are going to talk about here is the history of our knowledge of the law of attraction. When did humans first start realizing they were creating their own realities with thoughts?

Buddha was born in 623 BC and was a spiritual leader who founded Buddhism. He said, "*All that we are is the result of what we have thought.*" In Christianity, Judaism and Islam, Abraham plays an important part. He is referenced in biblical texts as saying that everything is brought to a person by a powerful universal law of attraction, whether good or bad, wanted, or unwanted.

The first time the term law of attraction was used in modern times to explain the idea that like attracts like was in 1877.

Helena Petrovna Blavatsky wrote and spoke about it as she traveled several European countries as a spiritualist and philosopher. Author Prentice Mulford is often credited as the first person to outline many of the principles of the law of attraction in 1886.

William Walker Atkinson wrote "Thought Vibration or the Law of Attraction in the Thought World" in 1906. This was followed using the term in the writings of Irish/American spiritualist William Quan Judge in 1915, and British socialist and women's rights activist Annie Besant in 1919. As communications technology improved, the law of attraction became something that was recognized globally in the early 20th century.

When the law of attraction really took off was when the aforementioned Jerry and Esther Hicks released nine books collectively titled as "The Teachings of Abraham". They explained in detail how this natural law works, and more importantly, how you can harness it to manifest whatever you desire.

Rhonda Bryne published the international bestseller "The Secret" in 2006. In it she speaks of the power of positive thinking and the law of attraction for creating your dream existence. That book and the subsequent film of the same name probably did more than any other single piece of media to turn the law of attraction into a common household term.

5 Ways Science Proves and Supports the Law of Attraction

People believe all kinds of things especially with the advent of the internet and conspiracy theories, anything can seem possible to us. There are individuals that are certain Bigfoot, the Loch Ness monster and the Yeti are real animals. They may very well be, or they may be some type of animal/human hybrid. However, to this point, the existence of those three cryptids has not been proven.

We mention this to illustrate that sometimes it is nice to have science and factual evidence to back up your belief. For those people that do not believe in the law of attraction, there are several ways science has established this natural law exists. Here are just 5 of the many scientific proofs of the LOA.

1 – 1984 Research of Physicist Dr. John Wheeler

Dr. Wheeler has suggested that for our universe to exist, something had to observe it. The observation led to the creation of the universe, and even shaped how and why it existed. He decided to test his theory on a more manageable scale.

His 1984 experiment on the observation of particles suggests that the law of attraction does indeed exist.

We will summarize his research without going into a bunch of scientific jargon. When he and his team consciously observed particles, it changed the state of the particles. Not only did it change what was happening, but also how that particle got to the point where it was being observed.

This indicates that observing something can change what it does and how it exists right now. Furthermore, it offers some groundbreaking evidence that current observations change the activity of a particle in the past. In other words, your observation led the particle to being observed by you in the first place.

The law of attraction states that whatever you give your focused attention to, will become a reality. You are literally changing what happened in the past so that your current situation is what you desire. Like with the particles in Wheeler's research, your observation and attention change your present reality.

You can manifest what you think about.

2 – 2007 Study Reported in the Yonsei Medical Journal

Ji Young Jung is a Korean researcher that worked with his colleagues to study the effect of positive thinking on a person's life. You have probably had someone tell you that positive thinking leads to positive results or to always look on the bright side of life. This idea mirrors the premise that you can use the law of attraction to create a positive reality rather than a negative situation.

What the researchers found was that positive thinking correlated with more "life satisfaction". Study participants that were more positive and upbeat tended to be happier with their lives. The researchers suggested that this is proof that positive thinking exercises can increase the likelihood that you can manifest the type of life you desire.

Here is a statement made by the researchers about the study:

"These findings offer promise of positive thinking as an approach for psychological interventions designed to promote life satisfaction."

That is powerful stuff. It shows how conscious human thought can lead to psychological processes that make a person more likely to enjoy his life. People enjoy positive aspects of their existence more than negative aspects.

Simply put, focusing energy on positive thoughts can create a positive reality. Being happy and thinking positive thoughts really does improve mood and our ability to face what life throws at us head on. Try it!

3 – Mirror Neuron Research

This is another piece of substantial scientific research that argues you can live a life by design. You can design your life rather than having to exist in a reality where you have no control. Mirror neurons were discovered in the 1990s, so they are a recent finding for neurologists.

Some Italian scientists noticed that a specific set of neurons acted a certain way when a macaque monkey grabbed some type of object. This in and of itself was no major discovery. Your nervous system drives your behavior and is also influenced by your actions. However, what was unique here is that this same set of neurons was discovered when the monkey saw some other primates grab the same object that he did.

These nerve cells were given the name mirror neurons because of this mirrorlike trait.

Because of recent research (the first couple of decades of the 21st century), we know mirror neurons explain how we attract certain energies. In humans, just like in the macaque monkey research, these nerve cells fire and transmit energy when we perform an action or observe that same action being performed by someone else.

The person that is merely observing an action is much more likely to perform that action than if the observation had not been made. Monkey see, monkey do.

This supports the law of attraction. If you act kind, happy and positive, you are going to trigger those actions in others that observe you. You are attracting behaviors that you see as positive. This can be demonstrated when people who are happy and fun to be around get invited out more often or to more parties. Or indeed have a bigger social circle.

However, remember that the law of attraction works to deliver negative or positive results. So, if your thoughts, energies, and efforts are negative in nature, you will attract a negative experience. If you are constantly angry, mean, and unsuccessful, that is the reality you will see around you.

4 – Science Proves Visualization Does Influence Reality

Visualization is a big part of harnessing the law of attraction to your benefit. Visualization is a combination of mental focus, attention, and energy, the three defining components of LOA according to Michael Losier.

Multiple neurological studies have shown that visualization triggers activity in specific parts of your brain. As you visualize a desired outcome, those brain regions respond in the same way as they would as if you were taking actions that led to the outcome.

Additionally, the human brain appears to get bored and takes little to no action when you verbalize what you want. Researchers are still not sure why this happens. If you instead visualize or draw what it is that you want, the brain wakes up and responds with a much deeper sense of interest and focus.

Incredibly, this leads your brain to store the memory of what you have visualized as something you have already done, whether or not it has happened yet.

Your attention, perception, memory, motor control and planning are all affected by visualization. Your brain is being trained to create a visualized reality. You are more likely to manifest the things you want and the life you want to have when you supply yourself with mental imagery of what it is you desire. We believe that visualizations have tangible benefits in realizing goals and aspirations.

5 – Affirmations Work to Create a Desired Reality

Affirmations are used in a law of attraction practice. Once again, science steps in to prove that this can help you achieve goals and create a positive reality. One study out of the University of Exeter agrees with other research in this regard.

The Exeter researchers studied the influence of "constructive repetitive thought" on future outcomes. They wanted to see if it was possible to program the human brain for a desirable set of circumstances rather than merely hoping those circumstances would develop. The research showed that the study participants who regularly and consistently told themselves they could accomplish something were more likely than others to be successful. This could of course be because people who were studied are more driven, but the evidence suggests otherwise.

The fact that affirmations are used by therapists to help clients recover from trauma and depression is further proof that this law of attraction practice can shape reality.

How the Law of Attraction Works

Like things are attracted to each other because everything is composed of energy. This is a belief common to many ancient spiritual practices and religions across the world. The belief in traditional Chinese culture that a vital energy force is in every living thing goes back many thousands of years. In ancient Indian spiritual practices, there is also a belief that there is energy in all things.

This was not widely accepted in the Western world until proven by scientists the 20th century.

Quantum physics explained that there is no such thing as solid matter in our universe. You are not made of solid parts. This is tough to understand and a very strange concept, but it has to do with the fact that everything is made up of atoms. As it turns out, atoms are not solid, physical things. They are made up of three subatomic particles: proteins, electrons, and neutrons. Electrons travel so quickly that they do not inhabit a physical space for very long.

Additionally, atoms have been scientifically proven to be 99.99% space. They have no physical structure. They are energy units. Since everything is made up of atoms and atoms are nothing more than energy, everything is essentially energy. The smartphone you can't live without and look at frequently, the garden at your home, the clouds in the sky, you, your friends and the vehicle you drive are nothing more than collections of fluid energy.

As Nobel prize-winning physicist Niels Bohr said, *"Everything we call real is made up of things that cannot be regarded as real."*

The Role of Vibration in the Law of Attraction

Since everything in the universe is energy and energy are constantly vibrating, you are going to have energy fields influencing each other. This is the way the law of attraction works. If your energy state is operating at the same frequency as chocolate, you will find yourself drawn to chocolate and it will be drawn to you. It sounds crazy but it is true.

Perhaps you have recently thought about a friend you have not been in contact with for years. Why are you thinking about that person so often now? The answer is that the two of you are giving off the same energy frequency. Before you know it, if the two of you stay tuned to each other's energy, you will receive a call from that person. Think about how many times this has happened? Scary isn't it? Maybe you randomly bump into him on the street, or you will take the time to reach out to him.

Here is a simple example of like energies attracting each other that happens to a lot of people.

You hear a song that you really like on the radio. You sing along with the song as it plays, and it gets you in a good mood. When you are happy as opposed to sad, full of joy and happiness rather than frustration and anger, your nervous system takes notice. It begins to influence your energy so that you vibrate at the frequency of the music you love. You become enveloped by joy and happiness.

Before you know it, you are hearing that song everywhere. You are drawn to it, and it's being drawn to you. What then happens is you think about this song at some time in the future and then it pops up on the radio again. I bet this has happened more than once too!

As we mentioned earlier, this can work to your disadvantage. If your energy vibrates at a frequency range that is like that of drugs or alcohol, guess what you are going to crave, even if you are not physically addicted. You may wonder why you always seem to attract the wrong kind of partner too. You seem destined for unhealthy relationships that are unfulfilling and maybe even dangerous.

The fact is that you truly are attracting that undesirable type of partner and you always will ... until you change the frequency range of your energy. That's right, you can change how your energy vibrates so that you attract the things you want.

To recap, here are some law of attraction truths:

- All things are energy.

- Energy vibrates at certain frequencies.

- Similar frequencies are attracted to each other because they are aligned.

- You can change your energy's vibrational frequencies to attract what you want.

Next up we discuss why you might be drawing negative experiences to yourself. As much as we can and want to attraction positive energies, we can also attract negative energies too. You will also discover how to stop fostering belief systems that are attracting anything less than favorable outcomes.

How Limiting Beliefs Attract the Opposite of What You Want

Limiting beliefs will inevitably hold you back. They keep you from creating the dream reality you have always desired. When you think about it, this does not make a lot of sense at face value. Why would someone continually foster beliefs that lead to negative consequences? The average person has belief systems that keep them from being everything they can be, but they also have thoughts of success and fulfillment and abundance.

Why do these limiting thought patterns seem to overpower healthier beliefs? Why is negativity so strong in the human mind?

One theory is when the brain is not occupied or busy it will always revert to negative thought patterns; this is a human default setting. So, to use an extreme example of this the following could be applied; Take two people, one is sitting on a yacht with a glass of champagne taking in the sun's rays. Another is working as a cleaner and is cleaning a toilet. Who is the happier? All of us will always suggest it the person lying on the yacht sipping a drink and sunbathing. However, if we go back to what we have just discussed, and it is true that an unoccupied mind will always revert to negative thoughts then we would be wrong.

The person cleaning the toilets would be therefore the happier at the time, their mind would be focused solely on what they are doing and not thinking about what disasters cold befall them. On the other hand, the person on the yacht with nothing else to think about will inevitably start thinking about what could go wrong to disturb their leisure.

One of the reasons which has been proven by science is that many people inherit negative behavior patterns and thought systems from previous generations. The opposite can also be true. Your past generations may have developed values and ideas that lead to wonderful and positive realities that you have also inherited.

This is often the case with people that can't seem to do anything wrong. This can frustrate you, because you try so hard to create a wonderful life and cannot, and these people seem to live a dream existence effortlessly and unconsciously. How can this be and what is the answer to this perceived dilemma?

The answer lies in genetics and has been proven using mice and cherry blossoms.

Brian Dias and his team of researchers at Emory University School of Medicine in Atlanta believed the experiences of previous ancestors influenced the physiological makeup of future generations. One possible example of this concerns people who lived through the Dutch famine of 1944.

Many of the survivors of that devastating famine went on to become parents. Their children had markedly lower birth weights and more health problems than what was the norm. That generation's children also had the same health issues. Could it be that the survivors of the famine equated their environment with that negative life experience and then passed that belief genetically to future generations?

Dias believed so. He and Dr. Kerry Ressler had mice smell cherry blossoms. While smelling that scent, the mice received slight but noticeable electric shocks. There were also mice in the experiment that were either exposed to some other scent, or no scent at all.

The cherry blossom mice mated. The new generation of mice was exposed to the cherry blossom scent for the first time. Even though they had no knowledge of the blossoms or the aroma they gave off, these young mice were supersensitive to the scent. They could detect it in extremely low quantities and would avoid it if possible. Mice born to the control group that did not undergo the cherry blossom conditioning responded normally to the aroma. It is basically how evolution works.

What is just as incredible is that the second-generation mice born to the first-generation offspring of the cherry blossom mice also inherited the genetic disposition to disliking the cherry blossom scent. The study was published in 2013 in the Nature Neuroscience journal.

The modifications which affect genetic makeup before birth are called epigenetic mechanisms. This simply means that an environment or experience can cause the attachment of certain chemicals to genes. This works as a warning system that is passed on to the genetic makeup of subsequent generations.

Studies were conducted to see if the mice communicated their negative experience to their offspring, and this was not the case. The mice conditioned to fear cherry blossoms showed higher levels of chemical receptors for the cherry blossom odor. In other words, this proved that the condition was passed through genetics, and not through communication or some other form of teaching.

This shows that limiting self-beliefs and fears can be genetically acquired. You can get them from your family tree. Fortunately, beliefs that are holding you back can be changed. You can embrace a belief in abundance and fulfillment, and then naturally pass this belief to your children while attracting the reality you desire. Just as much as we can impart fears and anxieties, we can also transfer positive emotions too.

How to Change Limiting Self-Beliefs with LOA

If you have a belief system which is creating a negative reality for you, it can be powerful and hard to step away from. As you just learned, this could be something that has been passed on through generations. Your genetic makeup believes that this is the only way the world operates. You unconsciously and automatically respond to certain environments, experiences or encounters because of the way you were hardwired. This can be detrimental to your health and happiness and ultimately your long-term future.

Sometimes we create unhealthy beliefs because we were exposed to some type of trauma as a child. Even as an adult, you respond with neutral, negative, or positive feelings to everything that happens to you. You have literally been hard wired to respond in negative ways and do this subconsciously.

When you are giving off negative vibrations because of something you have experienced, the universe begins to expose you to more of that type of experience. This explains why you seem to be stuck in a rut sometimes. No matter how hard you try, you can't get out of a cycle of negativity. A self-fulfilling prophecy if you like.

People sometimes live their entire lives without understanding how to change this unfortunate existence. After years of living this way, they just believe this is their lot in life and there is nothing they can do about it.

Nothing could be further from the truth though. You can change the frequency range at which your energy vibrates. This immediately and naturally changes what you will start attracting and realizing. You simply need to exert your will and focus your energy and attention to create a desirable physical reality that begins with the appropriate thoughts.

Understand that Beliefs Are Not Facts

Why is it that two people can have the same experience but believe entirely different things about that experience? It is simply because beliefs are not factual information. Beliefs are nothing more than what you think about a particular situation. The way you interpret events and circumstances, people, and things creates your belief system.

These are psychological marching orders that influence how your nervous system works. Your nervous system is largely responsible for the emotions you feel, and your emotions drive your actions for better or worse. Your actions and behaviors create your environment and experiences. This is how your beliefs lead to your reality.

There has probably been at least one point in your life where your beliefs were challenged. You learned that what you believed was incorrect. You were given powerful evidence that you were wrong, and this led to a new way of thinking. This can be the turning point in your life that your beliefs can be changed, and that they are not facts. We have a very powerful muscle called our brain and just as it can be hard wired to think in a certain way, we can also learn, listen, and ultimately train ourselves to change the way we think too.

This is the first important step to changing your current beliefs that are keeping you from manifesting a desired reality. Change how you think, and you can also change what happens to you.

Identify What You Want

It is not uncommon for a person to refuse to change his mind. This is because your belief systems are comfortable. You have led your life believing a certain way, and the thought of changing that belief can be scary. Stepping out of your belief comfort zone takes effort and many of us avoid extra effort. Why change anything if it is going to be hard work when you have convinced yourself you are happy?

What is going to happen if you think another way? Your comfortable, self-limiting beliefs have manifested your reality. Their energy frequency is unfortunately attracting a less than fulfilling situation for you. Even so, since your belief that you will never be wealthy has created a situation where you struggle financially, this reinforces that belief. Ultimately you settle for what you believe and do not make the extra effort in this example, to step out of your comfort zone and try and make more money.

How could any other reality be possible? You have tried in the past to overcome your financial troubles, to no avail. Because you expected financial ruin, that is what you got. You see this as a fulfillment of your belief, and your psychological makeup congratulates you for believing properly. "I told you so" is an often-repeated phrase that many people use

<u>The problem is that this is simply a belief and not a fact.</u>

What you believe to be factual is only your interpretation of the situation. Your belief can be changed, which changes your vibrational energy, and you can attract abundance and wealth rather than scarcity and financial problems.

The first thing you need to do before you can manifest a new reality is to look at your life and see what you want to change. The problem is that your stubborn, limiting self-beliefs do not want you to change your mind. They are happy just as they are. You are alive, so that is proof to your brain and nervous system that your current beliefs are healthy and positive.

Since it can be difficult to recognize ingrained beliefs that are limiting your life, do something that is much easier. Identify what it is you truly want. You are going to put your current belief systems to the side and instead clarify what you need to live your dream reality. To do so, ask yourself some form of the following questions.

- What is the first thing that comes to mind when I ask myself, *"What do I want more than anything else?"*

- What relationships would I like to have?

- What personal traits and characteristics would I like to possess? What behaviors or habits would I like to remove?

- What financial reality would be perfect? How long would I work? Would I work at all? What would I be doing? How much money do I need for my dream reality?

- What does my dream health look like?

- What goals would I like to achieve in all areas of my life? Divide them into short and long-term goals, but don't dream small.

- What is the underlying reason or reasons for these desires? Why do I want what I want? What are the benefits of these dream realities?

You may not care to change your physical health in any way. Your drive may be purely financial. The opposite might be true for you. Still, it is important to ask these types of questions in every aspect of your life. The more reasons you have for change, the greater the motivation. Write all your answers down, a visual guide of what you desire can have a positive outcome.

Speaking of motivation, dig deep when answering these questions. Telling yourself you want to be rich does not get to your real motivation for wealth. Keeping asking yourself WHY you want to achieve a certain goal. Go until you cannot find any deeper motivation.

Here is an example.

Let us say the first thing that comes to mind when you ask yourself what you want more than anything else is wealth. The next thing you should ask is why you want wealth. Your answer may be because your wealthy friends are always travelling, and you are envious of this ability. Why is this important to you? You answer that you have never been able to travel, and you admire people who can because you are always spellbound by their stories.

Now you are really getting down to the WHY of your desire to be wealthy. This is a powerful driving force in achieving what you desire.

It is important to keep this list as detailed as possible. Tell yourself you want to make $150,000 per year as a self-published author selling your books on Amazon's Kindle platform so people will respect you, rather than just saying you want to have a lot of money. Do you want to lose weight? That is not focused enough. Say that you want to drop 30 pounds in 90 days while building muscle, so you are ready for beach season. It is the specifics that will get you over the line quicker and keep you focused along the way.

Write your answers down and refer to them often to keep your energy heading in the right direction. Look at them daily.

Identify Your Self-Limiting Beliefs ... Here's How

You can fool yourself regarding which of your beliefs are healthy or unhealthy. You have held many of your self-limiting beliefs for a long time. This makes it difficult to change.

You can rationalize a negative belief system as a defense mechanism to keep you from changing. Therefore, it is important to look at your beliefs with your list of important goals in front of you. If a belief hampers your progress on your path to getting what you want, you must be honest with yourself and admit this is a limiting belief.

You will find that you were not aware consciously of many of the negative beliefs you have fostered. This is because they can hide beneath your conscious awareness. Fortunately, there are proven ways to unearth these hidden and limiting self-beliefs.

Look at what happens when you try to overcome a challenge. What is keeping you from conquering the problem? Many times, there is an unhealthy belief that is keeping you from succeeding. You previously believed this way of thinking was positive and helping you in some way. You need to recognize it as keeping you from attracting what you want. Limiting self-beliefs will sometimes present themselves as the following behaviors.

- You procrastinate instead of dealing with a situation. You prefer to put something off rather than make a decision. You can always get to it tomorrow.

- You will not do something unless you can do it perfectly. You believe your actions must be perfect, otherwise there is no need to do anything.

- When something negative happens, you tell yourself that happens all the time. This is just who you are, and these things always happen to you.

- Situations often make you think about your fears. You hesitate because your fear is holding you back.

- Your self-talk is negative. Your inner voice never sees the positive possibility in a situation, and instead expresses things in negative terms.

- You worry about the "what if" result of failure.

- You jump to negative conclusions even when there is not a lot of evidence that you should do so.

- Your knee-jerk reaction is to make an excuse.

- Complaining about your current life and how hard it is to make a new life is a constant behavior.

Now turn once again to the list of things you want. What is the first thought you have when you think of losing 25 pounds and getting ready for beach season? Do you immediately think that probably will not happen because you do not have enough time? This is nothing more than an excuse. The ability to attract the most amazing outcomes in your life is so powerful that you can achieve things you previously thought were impossible.

Do not let a self-limiting belief like excuse-making get your way. As you look through your goals and imagine starting out on a path to achieving them, list any beliefs that are trying to keep you from acting. These are beliefs which are unhealthy, and which are creating negative energy frequencies that are attracting the opposite of what you desire.

There are proven questions you can ask yourself to move limiting self-beliefs from your unconscious mind to conscious awareness. Ask these questions as you are considering your important goals.

- What makes me think this is going to be too difficult?

- What do I think will stop me?

- Am I making excuses instead of taking action?

- What did my self-talk just tell me? Did it use positive or negative language?

- Looking at this objectively, what do I think about this situation?

- What is the one thing holding me back from pursuing this dream reality?

- I am feeling resistance. Where is it coming from? What is the core emotion that is creating this resistance?

- Is my current fear of taking action coming from something I remember as a child? If so, is it still valid?

- If I could talk to the version of me that exists in my dream reality, what advice would he give me right now?

- If my knee-jerk reaction is to complain, is this really the healthiest behavior?

- Am I only believing this goal achievement is impossible because I have not realized it before?

Never forget that a belief is just an assumption. It is not a truth.

You can decide to believe anything about a situation or event. It is up to you to choose positive rather than negative beliefs. The series of questions we just covered can help you decide if your current beliefs are appropriate for a given situation.

You can feel very uncomfortable when you consider changing beliefs or values you have held for possibly your entire life. Just because a belief is long held does not mean it is helping you. If your current reality is something you want to change, you are going to have to change your beliefs and actions.

The definition of insanity is to expect a different set of results while continuing to do the same thing as you have in the past. Successful implementation of the law of attraction to manifest what you want in life requires that you ditch self-limiting beliefs and create belief patterns that attract the life you know you deserve.

7 Myths and Misconceptions of LOA You Need to Dismiss

Before we go any further, we need to clear up some rumors and misconceptions about the law of attraction. You may have encountered these thoughts in the warnings of others. Perhaps you share some of these beliefs too. For LOA to manifest what you want there can be no halfway buy-in. Your energy will reflect that, and your vibrational frequencies will not be aligned with the things you want.

Avoid believing the following half-truths and falsehoods for total belief in the powerful law of attraction at work in the universe.

1 - LOA is Magical!

Try this. Imagine what you want. Make a positive statement about it. See yourself owning your dream reality. Now do not waste another minute worrying about achieving this goal. What happened? Most likely ... absolutely nothing.

This is not "say a magic word and your dream will be realized" smoke and mirrors. Your best possible existence will not be handed to you magically with no effort on your part. You are not experiencing the misdirection of a stage magician that uses trap doors and other props to give you the appearance of a reality that really isn't there. You will not be handed your dream existence on a silver platter because of some supernatural manifestation. Thinking alone without some form of action will simply be not enough.

This is a natural process. The law of attraction is working right now in your life, attracting the things to you that vibrate at your same energy level and frequency.

Sure, when you begin visualizing, using affirmations, meditating and going through the manifestation process we will share with you in a bit, it may seem magical that you begin to receive the things you want. However, there is no magic involved. Magic does not exist. The law of attraction does exist, and you just need to send that law in the right direction to realize the physical, emotional, financial, and spiritual rewards you are looking for.

<u>2 - The Law of Attraction Can't Be Proven by Science</u>

We need to bring this up again, even though we covered it in an earlier chapter. We have already shared with you 5 examples of how science has proven that the law of attraction exists in the natural world. Those are not the only pieces of research that support the idea that you are constantly attracting energy.

Think about it this way.

The propane or natural gas which powers products in your home is invisible. Natural gas does not even have a smell, so a detectable odor is added to it so you will know when you have a gas leak. Just because you cannot see this gas and, in some cases, cannot even smell it does not mean it cannot kill you. The law of attraction works the same way.

Just because you cannot see the vibrational energy that all things give off does not mean it isn't there. You do not need to understand the law of attraction or be able to touch it, feel it or see it for it to work. Electricity is invisible but if you were to stick your finger in a light socket, it would let you know it is there. LOA has been scientifically proven, and that is a good thing. That means your belief in this powerful, natural law can grow stronger because you know it exists. We just need to harness it.

3 - LOA Doesn't Work

This is one of the biggest myths you will hear about the law of attraction. Because its invisible, many people do not believe it can work. Those same people breathe invisible, odorless, and tasteless oxygen that keeps them alive every day, but they will tell you since they can't see, smell, or hear LOA, it can't be a real thing.

If it does not exist in their eyes, how can it work?

When you begin embracing the law of abundance, thinking positively, and keeping your vibrations high, you will start to see LOA working in your life. When you consistently work through the 5 steps needed for you to manifest what you want (don't worry, we cover this later), you will have no doubt that like energies attract each other.

Just as the law of gravity was working long before Newton explained it, LOA has been around forever. As long as the natural world has been in existence, similar energy frequencies have been attracted. You may as well say that the sun is not very hot, because that isn't true either.

<u>4 - LOA Requires too Much Effort</u>

Some people will tell you the law of attraction is hard to get to grips with and therefore not worth the effort to pursue. It is not hard at all. It does all the work. All you must do is get your energy right. If you are just learning to use the law of attraction to push your desires towards you, there will be some work involved learning how to control your thoughts.

Soon enough, the process begins to work on its own. You learn to act and think in a way that focuses your energy and intent so that the things you desire are magnetized and pulled towards you.

If you think LOA requires too much effort, consider your present reality. How long have you been banging your head up against the wall to try to get the things you desire? How many years or decades have you lived a life that is a watered-down version of what you know you deserve? You have probably spent tireless hours of hard work for a long time trying to create your dream reality ... yet still you are not where you want to be. A poor negative mindset is restrictive and is evident in many people's lives.

Remember earlier where we mentioned your mind can make excuses for you to bailout on your journey to manifesting what you desire? This is nothing more than an excuse, a self-limiting belief.

5 - The Law of Attraction Is Based on Self-Centered and Greedy Desires

Some people believe the pursuit of money is evil. They may tell you that the Bible says, "Money is the root of all evil." That is incorrect. The Bible says, "The love of money is the root of all evil."

Wanting money is not a bad thing. Wanting abundance in any form is not bad either. What you do with the abundance that the law of attraction delivers to you is up to you. You can certainly use your newfound wealth, health, intelligence, influence, or possessions to do bad things. That is your choice. What you will find with the law of attraction is that when you begin to act in a manner which is negative in the eyes of the universe, all you will attract from that point on is negative energy. This is not up for debate; it is a fact.

On the contrary, the law of attraction is not based on helping greedy and self-centered people. Those are negative emotions and energies. They will only attract negative results and outcomes. Besides, is wanting a fulfilled, happy, and rewarding life self-centered and greedy? Is it wrong that you want to finally live in harmony with the person you were intended to be? Of course, it is not. The people that tell you LOA is for greedy, self-centered people either do not know what they are talking about, or they do not want to see you succeed.

6 - You Can't Practice LOA If You Have Certain Religious Beliefs

We will say it again. The law of attraction is natural. There is no witchcraft or voodoo involved.

This is not a supernatural or magical undertaking. Whether you practice a specific religion or not, or you consider yourself a spiritual being of some type, LOA does not care. It does not have an opinion. It sees you as a natural being because you are truly a product of nature. It detects your energy and wants to attract similar energies to you because that is what makes sense to nature.

Would your religion tell you that the stars in the heavens, the trees and the mountains, the oceans and the deserts are off-limits? Surely, they would not. They tell you these are beautiful things created by nature and they are gifts you should appreciate. The law of attraction is the same thing, a natural gift that is already working in your life, so it only makes sense to get it working for you rather than against you.

Incidentally, when you start living a life of harmony with the universe, your appreciation of your spirituality or religion can only become greater.

7 - Law of Attraction is Not for Everyone

You should imagine the law of attraction as being totally objective. It does not have an opinion about you or anyone else. It does not have anything to say about rocks or trees or cars or money or wealth or health or the 20 pounds you want to lose.

It works for everyone and everything that gives off energy, automatically and with no judgment.

It is as natural and uncaring as a fire. If you burn your hand on a flame, it is not because the fire does not like you. Any person that walks up to that fire and sticks their hand in is going to receive the same burning experience. Gravity works for everyone, fire can burn or provide heat and illumination for everyone, and LOA works for everyone as well.

Embrace the Law of Abundance

To this point you have discovered that the way you think is the way you live. Master salesman, speaker and personal coach Jim Rohn was famous for saying something along these lines. He frequently told his students that they would become what they thought about most of the time.

Neurologists will tell you that you move towards your most predominant thought. Your brain finds it exceedingly difficult to focus on two things at once, so whatever it is that you think about most of the time, your brain prioritizes that.

If you decide that the universe believes in scarcity, that is what you are going to see. We move to our most predominant thoughts, so when we think that there isn't enough to go around, that someone has to lose something for someone else to win it, that is what we will magically see happening everywhere we go.

Of course, you could decide to embrace the opposite possibility. The choice is yours. You might want to develop the mindset that the universe has more than enough for everyone, and that if every person got what they wanted and they desired more, the universe would be happy to increase its abundance.

Think about the age-old question regarding your perception of a glass of water.

Imagine you have a glass container which holds 16 ounces of water at its fullest point. When it is bone dry it has 0 ounces of water in it. If there are 8 ounces of water in that container, is it half full or is it half empty? This is a philosophical question that quickly reveals whether you are a positive or negative thinker.

It also shows that in a split second you can decide to change how you look at anything. You can move from being a negative thinker (the glass is half empty) to be a positive thinker (the glass is halfway to being full). Remember, the law of attraction will align you with your beliefs because your beliefs have certain energy frequencies attached to them.

When you know for certain that there is limitless abundance in the universe, you begin to move towards that abundance and it begins to move towards you, thanks to the law of attraction.

Embrace this belief to the point where there is no way you would question it. By the way, abundance does not just mean limitless financial resources. You can seek abundance in any area of your life, using it to improve your relationships, your physical health, or anything else you want to change. It truly is amazing and even just the smallest of changes can have a massive impact on your quality of life.

Learn to Think Positively

Every seasoned LOA devotee will tell you how important it is to think positively. This cannot be overstated. Your outlook on life is everything. As with the example just mentioned, you can look at something negatively or positively. The negative person sees a half empty glass, and the positive thinker sees a glass that is half full.

Thinking positively is essential for you to use the law of attraction to manifest the reality you desire. It also has a positive impact on your mental wellbeing.

You can decide that you don't have enough money to pay your bills. You may instead tell yourself that you are so close to having all the money you need to pay your bills. The positive energy you put off when you consciously decide to adopt a positive viewpoint leads to higher vibrations. Negative energy and a negative outlook mean lower energy frequency levels. The higher you can get your vibrations the better, and we will discuss this in-depth in the next chapter.

If you do not believe in the power of positive thinking, then why do placebos work?

What are placebos? A placebo is a "dummy pill" that contains no active drugs or medicines. It works just like a medication for many people. There have been countless studies performed that display the power of the human mind to heal the body, and placebos prove that ability. The thought of taking a cure tricks the mind into thinking the body is getting better even if the cure has no actual true benefits.

A researcher will give two groups of people either a placebo or an actual medicine. Everyone in the study will have the same condition, such as an upset stomach, back pain or some other symptom related to the brain and nervous system. Incredibly, many people that receive placebos (dummy pills with no medicine) rather than real medicine will begin to get better!

This works time and again because the person taking the placebo believes it is medicine. They have taken medicine before and it has delivered the desired result, so their brain tells them they are not feeling any more pain or discomfort. This is a powerful example of how positive thinking can align your energy with the positive outcome you are looking for. If the brain can trick itself into thinking you are cured by taking a fake pill, then the mind can perform other more powerful tricks and this is where the positive energy of the law of attraction comes into its own.

The Importance of Keeping Your Vibrations High

Think about your energy as a radio wave signal. If you do not give off much of a signal, whatever you are broadcasting is not terribly noticeable. The more strength you give that signal, the further it can reach. The law of attraction works in a similar way. The higher you elevate your energy levels, the more access you have to the universe.

As it turns out, energy that vibrates at low frequencies is associated with scarcity, fear, self-loathing, failure, and other negative realities. When your energy vibrates at a high level, you access abundance, success, happiness, health, wealth, and other positive realities. Therefore, it is important to keep your vibrations high.

How do you do this? Two words ... get happy.

Do something that makes you smile every day, a few times a day if you can. Embrace happiness more than sadness. Make others laugh and feel happy, because it is a wonderful contagion, it spreads rapidly.

Experiencing positive emotions is a simple but amazingly effective way of keeping your vibrations high. This aligns you with the positive energy in the universe, which is where your desires and the things you want are going to be found.

By the way, you need to experience clean and positive happiness. If you feel a dark joy when you see a friend fail, this is not the happiness you are seeking. You should only feel empathy, sympathy, and a desire to help your friend if she stumbles and falls on life's journey. The happiness you want to seek out is that pure and clean joy you feel when you hug someone you care about and haven't seen for a long time.

Watch a smiling, laughing baby. Play with your children or grandchildren. Maybe you are genuinely happy when you are digging in your garden or taking a hike. Perhaps real joy comes to your heart when you give your spare time to a charitable organization. Whatever gives you clean and positive happiness, do it, and do it often. This will keep your energy vibrating at a high level and will give you the best opportunity to attract positive change in your life.

Express Gratitude Daily

Did you know that you give your health a boost when you express gratitude? It is true. People who are grateful for the blessings in their lives no matter how small and the things they have, live longer, healthier, and happier lives than those who do not.

This is because gratitude is telling the universe that you are thankful.

This is a positive statement. You have just learned how important positive thinking is and how universal energy rewards a positive mindset. Again, this is a simple choice. You can decide right now to focus your energy on the positive, wonderful things in your life, or the failures and shortcomings.

Start recording your thoughts in a daily gratitude journal. If you cannot carry it with you throughout the day, make sure you jot down daily experiences that you are grateful for. Then enter them into your journal each night. Read over them before you go to bed and the first thing in the morning. You might be amazed at how much peace and happiness this gives you.

You will find that when you express gratitude regularly, you become more giving. Gratitude is linked to abundance. When you are grateful for what you have you are more likely to give to others in some way. The universe sees this and figures that if you are capable of giving something, you must have an abundance of it.

What is the Law of Attraction except for like things attracting like things?

Your gratitude leads you to help others and give things to them that they need, and this instantly attracts abundance to you. Besides, studies tell us that grateful people enjoy less stress, anxiety, and depression than others. There are a lot of good reasons to practice gratitude daily.

The Problem with "The Secret"

We introduced the film and book "The Secret" when covering Law of Attraction history. The book's author should be commended because she has opened the eyes of millions around the world to the power of the law of attraction. The downside is that the book stops short of telling you exactly what you need to do to manifest the things you desire. It basically says that if you are always thinking positively then you will have everything you need.

This report goes step-by-step through just what you need to do to manifest your desires. There is a lot more to it than just having a positive mindset and wishing that you had something. Those are two important steps on the path to harnessing the power of LOA. However, as you can tell if you have read this far, there is much more that is required to sync your energy with the energy of the things you want in your life.

"The Secret" has a great message but stops short on substance. The reason why we mention this is that many people have become frustrated with the law of attraction since they purchased this book or saw the movie. They went home and thought positively about the things they wanted and received little to no positive results.

If this was you, we can understand your frustration.

As you are about to find out, one important step to manifesting what you desire with the Law of Attraction is acting. You must do everything we have talked about up to this point. This puts your mind and energy in the right place for you to attract what you want. Unfortunately, many people who read "The Secret" went home, sat down on their sofas, practiced positive thinking, and waited for their dreams to be realized. This clearly is not going to work.

This led to disappointment most of the time. That's because giving your attention to what you desire is not enough to convince the universe that your energy is worthy of attracting the energy of your dream reality. Remember from our earlier definition of the law of Attraction that you will attract "... whatever you give your attention, energy, and focus to."

You are naturally vibrating at some energy level all the time. With LOA, there is another type of energy that you need to harness, and that is action. When you fully buy into the natural process that is working here, your attention and desire can't help but lead you to taking focused and energetic action that will draw your desired reality to you like a magnet.

"The secret" is a wonderful book and has helped millions begin their journey to understanding the Law of Attraction. Its shortcoming is that it only highlights one important step in the manifestation process. What are the detailed steps that have worked for so many people to help the law of attraction manifest what they desire? Let us take a look.

5 Steps to Manifest Whatever You Desire with LOA

All your reading so far has brought you to this especially important point. It is highly recommended that you totally embrace what you have learned thus far. The manifestation of the things and experiences you desire comes more quickly when you are totally immersed in a law of attraction belief.

Go back over previous sections where you did not understand something or were not totally committed. Tell yourself that the more understanding and belief you have, the more positively powerful the Law of Attraction can be in your life. Then when you are ready to begin attracting the people, things and experiences you desire, then here are the 5 steps which have been proven to do exactly that.

1 - Give Yourself a Very Specific Target

Earlier you made a list of the things you want in life. You explored the emotions behind your desires and listed limiting beliefs that may be stopping you from achieving goals and realizing your dreams. Look at both of those lists again. Choose one of the things you want to manifest in your life.

Make sure it is one of your biggest desires.

Now look at the list of self-limiting beliefs. The fact that you wrote them down means you understand they are simply your opinions, and not facts. That means you can change them. You do not have to think this way. With that in mind, write down what it is you want to manifest and be very detailed.

Do not be vague. Write exactly what it is you want. If it is a new car, what color is it? What types of features and accessories does it have? Is it a convertible or hardtop? What does the interior look like and are the seats leather or cloth? How much does it cost?

The more details you use here, the better the chance that you will be able to realize your desire. This is because your energy is extremely focused, it is not vague, you have a target to reach out to. If you just write down that you want a new car, that doesn't give the law of attraction enough direction.

Different cars have different energy frequencies, so the universe doesn't understand what energy to send your way.

In this example, what are the emotions tied to your desire for this vehicle? Would you like to have it because it will turn heads and get you noticed? If so, focus on those thoughts as you write down the detailed description of your vehicle. Perhaps you drive a gas guzzler now and your dream car is a hybrid electric/gas model that is very efficient with fuel. If that is your reason for wanting this particular car, think about that and write it down with the description.

Make sure you have pen or pencil to hand and write on paper or in a journal. It is okay to keep a digital version on your smartphone or computer if you like, but make sure you have a handwritten copy as well.

Forbes magazine reported how much of a difference writing down your goals makes as far as achieving them goes. In an April 16 blog post, Forbes cited research that shows you are 20% to 40% more likely to achieve a goal when it was written down and vividly described.

Remember that people attract whatever they give their energy, attention and focus to. The more detailed and specific your goal is, the more laser-focused your attention and energy can be. You are putting out a very specific energy. Refer to this daily. Read it to yourself at least every morning and every night, if not more frequently. This ensures you keep your energy focused in the right direction.

2 - Visualize Already Having Achieved Your Dreams

We spoke earlier about how visualization has been scientifically proven to boost a person's goal achievement success rate. This is the second step in the manifestation process. You want to see what it is you desire in your mind's eye. In the previous step you wrote an extremely detailed description of what it is you want. Now you understand why it is so important to be detailed rather than vague. It makes the visualization process much easier.

Too many times when people try to create a mental visual image of something, they just think about what it looks like. That is certainly important too. Your eyes convey a lot of information to your brain. Vision is usually the first sense you use to gather information about your environment. The word visualization even has the word "visual" in it.

What you do not want to do is focus on just this one sense.

You have 5 senses – sight, smell, touch, hearing and taste. Get as many of them involved as you can. Can you smell what it is that you desire? Is it possible to taste it? What does it sound like? What does it feel like?

The more of your 5 senses you can be involved in this visualization process, the better it is for you. Your senses are strongly tuned to your emotions. This means the "why" is clearer when you attach all your senses to the visualization process because you make an emotional investment.

Now we are going to share something with you that very few people do when they visualize what it is, they desire. This is a powerful step that even some veteran Law of Attraction practitioners do not know. You want to look at what it is you desire from several different angles.

This is known as multi-perspective visualization.

Do not just visualize it from your viewpoint. How do other people look at it? If it is a physical object, what would other people say about it? Can they hear it, touch it, taste it, smell it? If your goal is to change a character trait, something you cannot touch and feel, how will people look at you when you have this trait or skill? What will they feel about you differently?

Now step outside of your body and look at yourself. Pretend you are someone who is seeing you after you have manifested what it is you desire. This third-person point of view is often used by professional athletes to improve their abilities.

To make this visualization process even more powerful, how about creating a dream board? This is a physical poster board, corkboard, or some other platform where you post pictures of what it is you desire. Now your visualization is not just in your mind. You can see it clearly with your own two eyes. Keep your dream board in a place where you see it every day. If you can make a duplicate dream board and keep it at work as well as at home, this gives you a double dose of motivation.

3 – Use Affirmations to Empower Your Subconscious

What are affirmations? They are conversations you have with yourself. By the way, you already make affirmations all the time, you just might not know you do it. Any time you talk to yourself out loud or in your mind silently, you are affirming something. You are making an affirmation.

Affirmations are incredibly powerful because of something called the reticular activating system (RAS).

This is a part of your brain that stands up and takes notice when you repeat something over and over. Your brain quickly notices thought patterns, words, and phrases when they are repeated. Your RAS instantly assumes that you would not be saying this time and time again unless it was important. Accordingly, your brain prioritizes this information. Therefore, you must be incredibly careful about what you tell yourself, either out loud or silently with your inner voice.

If you are looking for a definition, you can consider affirmations as positive sentences that you repeat to yourself that create belief in your subconscious mind.

It is your subconscious mind that diligently goes to work solving problems and pursuing your goals. It does it behind-the-scenes, while you are sleeping, working, and playing. Since your subconscious tirelessly works towards creating the reality of your affirmations, doesn't it make sense to make them positive rather than negative?

If you are like most people, you might be making damaging affirmations without realizing you are doing it. If you make a mistake do not say, "I always do that." Instead, tell yourself, "I am getting better at getting this right."

For the most powerful affirmations, they should be positive and in the present tense. Here are a few Law of Attraction affirmations that can help you manifest what you desire.

- I believe in myself and my abilities.

- I am talented in so many ways.

- I wake up each morning with gratitude for my wonderful life.

- I am a magnet to abundance and prosperity.

- I appreciate what I have, and I am attracting more abundance each day.

- My dreams are becoming reality right before my eyes.

- I visualize the way I want my life to be and it becomes that way.

- The universe constantly attracts (money, healthy relationships, success, etc.) to me.

- Anywhere I look, I see multiple opportunities to bring more (fill in the blank) into my life.

You do so many things in the morning to get you prepared for your day. One thing you should do is repeat affirmations to yourself. Say them out loud and not just silently. Embrace them. Attach your emotions to them. Make affirmations for every aspect of your life. Adopt the mindset that you absolutely believe these affirmations to be correct, and that you are not simply stating facts.

How you think affects your life in so many ways. Programming your subconscious to automatically begin creating the life you want with affirmations is a powerful thought process. Soon you will find that this process begins to change how you look at the world. You will stop seeing the glass as half empty and rather view it as half full. You see failures as opportunities, and simply events rather than a definition of who you are.

Write affirmations down and keep them with you. Pull them out and read them throughout your day whenever you need a mental boost. This will keep the universe well informed as to who you are and what you deserve. Believe us when we say this is a powerful method of changing your life for the better.

4 - Meditate

Meditation has been around a long time. It is an amazing stress reliever. You can literally feel stress leaving your body and mind within minutes or even seconds after you begin to meditate. The health benefits attached to meditation are many, and studies show that people who meditate regularly live longer, healthier, and happier lives than those who don't meditate at all.

Meditation began as a spiritual practice sometime between 3,500 and 5,000 BC. This is where we first find evidence of meditation on wall art found in India. Proof that meditation works in your life is easy to find.

Have you ever been having a rough day and you retreated to a quiet, calm place? You may have taken a few deep breaths and closed your eyes so you could clear your mind and focus your thoughts. You did not think about much of anything, but just enjoyed your quiet, peaceful environment.

Whether you knew it or not, you were meditating.

It really is that easy to meditate. One thing you want to change from a traditional meditation practice is what you are going to think about. Meditation usually has you focus on your breathing and nothing else. You don't think about anything. You just exist in the present moment. A living breathing human being.

For the best law of attraction benefits, you want to meditate while thinking about what it is you desire. Visualize it in your mind's eye. If you begin to get very emotional while in this process, take some time to calm your nerves. Your meditation should be peaceful and tranquil.

You can focus your vision on your dream board or simply close your eyes and think about what it is that you desire. Breathe deeply and slowly release your breath. Make sure you are in a peaceful and quiet environment with no distractions of any kind. You only need a few minutes of free time to meditate. You should prioritize time for meditation in your schedule because this is a vital step in the manifestation process. At the end of a working busy day is the perfect time to set some time aside to think, breath, and be.

<u>5 - Take Focused, Inspired Action with Attention and Energy</u>

Let us look again at Michael Losier's definition of the law of attraction.

"You attract whatever you give your attention, energy and focus to."

This fifth step of the law of attraction manifestation miracle is often overlooked. People say that the law of attraction did not work for them, and maybe it did not work the way they wanted it to for a particularly good reason. This is most likely to have happened because this fifth step was skipped.

When you visualize something, you have a strong desire for, you get the attention of the law of attraction. The same thing happens when you write down precisely what it is that you are looking for. Dream boards help focus your attention as we discussed earlier. Meditation and affirmations are important steps in the manifestation process as well.

When you do all these things and you truly embrace the idea that you can create your own physical reality by thinking it into existence, you cannot help but act. You feel so certain that you deserve your dream reality and that it is heading your way, and you want to do everything you can to make it happen.

You begin to feel that whenever you can take smart action that will attract your desired reality, you want to do exactly that.

Unfortunately, too many people expect the Law of Attraction to help them achieve their goals without them taking any voluntary action at all. That is not the way it works. Up to this point you have been doing everything to put your mind and your energy in alignment with your desires.

Now the universe will start sending you little clues that you need to act. It is after all how we get things done, if we start getting things done with a heart and head full of positive thoughts and vibrations, we are more likely to achieve our desired outcomes.

If you spontaneously feel that you should call someone, make that call. You may get a strong urge seemingly out of the blue to attend an event or to go someplace. These are signals you are receiving because your energy is becoming aligned with your dream reality. Do not turn a deaf ear to what your intuition is telling you. This is the universe pushing you closer to what it is that you want.

If you do not think you are receiving these intuitive messages, you can still take action.

You know the things you need to do to improve the odds that you will create the reality you want. If you want to manifest financial prosperity you are probably going to have to stop needlessly spending money. If you desperately desire to lose 15 pounds, maybe the action you should take is not eating a pizza with all the toppings right before bedtime.

You have focused your energy on what you want. Now it is time to turn that energy into action. Trust your instincts and take some actual steps towards what it is you desire, and the law of attraction will help you get it.

Conclusion

The law of attraction is already working in and around your life. It is going on out in the universe and finding a match for the energy you give off. This may not currently be creating the life of your dreams. If that is the case, understand that your dream life is only just around the corner. You simply need to change the energy you give off to change the results you are seeing in your life.

Start thinking more positively. Envision your dream reality. Frequently have a conversation with yourself about self-limiting beliefs and doubts which may be holding you back from creating the life of your dreams. The next time something bad happens to you or you hit a stumbling block on your life's journey, look at it positively rather than negatively. Learn from it and move on.

Any problem or difficulty can be seen as a wonderful opportunity with the right mindset. An education of sorts.

Meditate and use affirmations to attract what you want. There are plenty of good reasons why people have been meditating for thousands of years. This practice not only relieves stress and anxiety. It also focuses your energy and attention on the things you want out of life, making it easier for the universe to create that reality and manifest what you want. A healthy mind really does help the body stay fit and healthy.

You truly can attract what it is you desire whether it be a physical object, a skill or ability, a financial change, a better relationship, or anything else. Since the law of attraction is already working in your life, it makes sense to help it deliver positive rather than negative results. The information in this guide can help you do just that.

Before we finish lets just take one second to appreciate what we already have. Do not get too hung up on what you haven't got and what you desire. All of this can of course be obtained as we have read in the previous chapters but let us not also forget to appreciate all we already have. Do not be distracted by all the things you don't need. Focus on what is important to you.

Good luck, and here's to many happy and productive years.

A message from the Author

Hi, thank you purchasing my book. My name is Faye and I'm passionate about healthy, holistic living. Since I can remember I have had a keen interest as to what makes us tick as human beings and how we can improve our lives through positive healthy actions for both mind and body!

I'm also interested in healthy diets, eating and gardening. I especially love growing and foraging for organic foods. I have discovered it compliments my healthy lifestyle perfectly.

I grew in a large family and we shared many wonderful meals even on a modest budget. This has led me into looking at healthy affordable treatments and foods to maintain a wonderful healthy lifestyle.

Keeping fit physically is also a big part of my life, I particularly like running and walking. I guess this stems from my childhood spent running and walking the local fields with my brothers and sisters.

If you enjoyed this guide, then please find a little time to leave a review. It really means a lot and helps me reach more readers.

Thank you
Faye

<u>**More Books from The Author:**</u>

- <u>Aromatherapy: How to use natures remedies to improve your health and wellbeing</u>

- <u>Crystals: Crystal Healing for Beginners, Discover the Healing Power of Crystals and Minerals</u>

- <u>Natural Remedies: A Guide to Preparing and Using Plants & Herbs to Heal Your Body & Mind</u>

- <u>Meditation: A Guide to Using Meditation to Enhance Your Life, Health and General Well-being</u>

- <u>Happiness: 12 Habits of Really Happy People & How They Can Work for You</u>

- <u>Healing: 3 Book Collection (Aromatherapy, Crystals, and Natural Remedies)</u>